MW01281876

Copyright © 2018 by Roberta Tabb
All rights reserved.

This book or any portion thereof may not be reproduced or used in any manner
whatsoever without the express written permission of the publisher except for
the use of brief quotations in a book review.

The advice and strategies found within may not be suitable for every situation.
This work is sold with the understanding that neither the author nor the publisher
is held responsible for the results accrued from the advice in this book.

Printed in the United States of America

ISBN-13: 978-1983540431
ISBN-10: 1983540439

Editing by Jennifer Fitzpatrick
Cover & Book design by Roberta Tabb

Roberta Tabb
www.therobertashow.com
www.simplytabbtastic.com

START.

**START, over & over again—
as many times as it takes.**

JUST START!

—Roberta Tabb

simply Tabbtastic

Prepare to Prep recommendation list

SINGLE SERVE BLENDER OR FOOD PROCESSOR
JUICER
WOODEN SKEWERS
SEALABLE PLASTIC BAGGIES
6 - 32 OUNCE MASON JARS
6 - 16 OUNCE MASON JARS
6 - 24 OUNCE STORAGE CONTAINERS
6 - 1 PINT STORAGE CONTAINERS

SIMPLYTABBTASTIC.COM | THEROBERTASHOW.COM

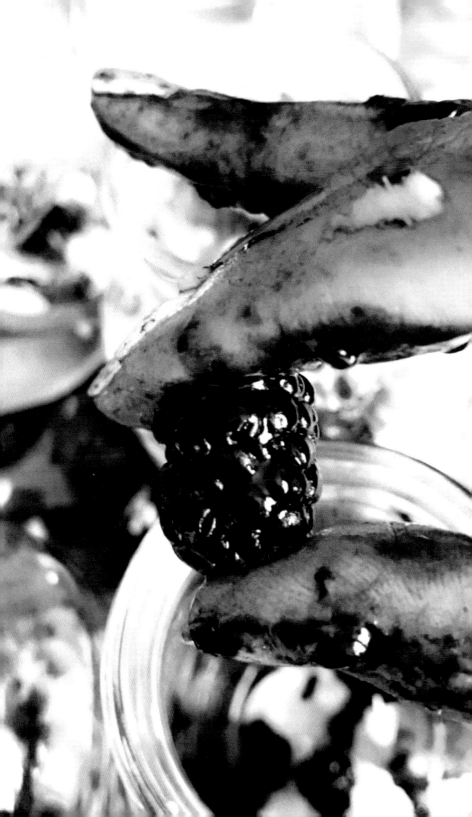

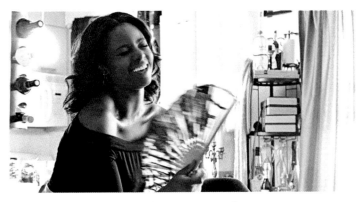

I created this simple guide for the same reason I created my blog...

To share a tangible source of relatable information for clean, healthy living. My life is not alchemy; it's a series of well-thought consistent routines. From (sometimes forced) daily positive thought patterns to weekly meal preps, consistency and dedication rule my being.

I'm a strong believer in simple food, but more so in REAL food. Most of the recipes I offer contain less than five ingredients, spices included. More importantly than the number of ingredients, all the recipe ingredients are raw and natural. I'm not offering a magical health solution that involves expensive foods that are unattainable to the ordinary grocery shopper, I'm offering SIMPLE, EASY and CLEAN ingredient pairings. This guide will teach you what I learned and unlearned, and show you that the simpler the better when prepping daily nourishing food for yourself or family.

I believe that food should not only nourish, but taste delicious as well. I can promise with a few (maybe drastic) changes, your taste buds and body will be satisfied. The easiest way to start this process is to acknowledge why you like the food you enjoy. What foods do you like and why? Is your food fixation on preparation, additives, or the actual base ingredients?

At the age of 20 I weighed almost 300 lbs. I was completely, hopelessly, helplessly depressed. Unlike now, the multitudes of self help information from various sources was not available. Also, my background didn't afford me any help - that required money or access. No one could help me, so by chance, I decided to help myself.

More than ten years later I'm still helping myself and hopefully many of you too. Sharing my story and inspiring from afar has held me accountable for my own progression. You can either be the flame or the reflection of it. **With so many people sharing my flame, how could I not stay LIT?**

Just when I thought I couldn't go any further, or that my fitness or weight loss journey was complete, I was pushed to find a new way to reinvent and better my physical and mental health. As told from me to you personally, here are a few recipes, tips and words of inspiration from a person who is (to this day) still struggling to be better than she was yesterday.

I'll keep it simple and easy – Simply Tabbtastic.

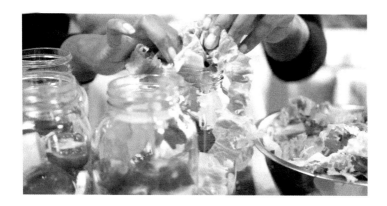

start

"Just Start" is my favorite piece of advice for anyone on the verge of a life change. Quick and dirty. It doesn't matter if it's Wednesday at 3:52 pm, or Saturday at 6pm - **START.** Tomorrow, Sunday, next month or at the beginning of the year is too far away to begin to change. If your serious about change START this instant. There are small things you can do this moment to begin the change. **TAKE ACTION:** Throw out junk foods, download a fitness app, create a healthy Pinterest board, do a set of lunges or jumping jacks, take a walk.

accountability

Throughout the process it will be YOU working against and with you. Day in and day out, you will find excuses to not push forward. Only you can account for your actions. **TAKE ACTION:** Write your fitness goals down, long and short term. Check them off the list when you hit them no matter how big or small. Goals can include meal prepping for the week, workout routines for the day, calorie tracking and water consumption.

inspiration

Inspiration is an overused word that is thrown around so often that it easily loses meaning - and yet I use it constantly. Once you find out what inspires you, it will take on a life of its own. My personal inspiration comes from believing in my own potential and visualizing the person I will become. **TAKE ACTION:** Look for your inspiration in everything: your family, your career, or a previous goal realized. Start by looking WITHIN. First and foremost, I am my own motivation and inspiration - I'm constantly trying to impress myself.

get real

Realistic goal setting. We have to be real with ourselves every single day. The first step is acknowledging that there is a problem. Once you accept that truth, develop a plan of action. The final step is following through (see **accountability**). The best way to set yourself up for failure is over promising - it can be detrimental to your progress. If you've had a hard time getting started, it probably isn't realistic that you will lose 20 lbs in one month. 5 lbs is a hardship at the very beginning and to create change you have to start changing; this never happens overnight. **TAKE ACTION:** Start with what you have and work for the best, those small things and consistent choices you make will start to create the bridge you need to cross WHILE you're building it.

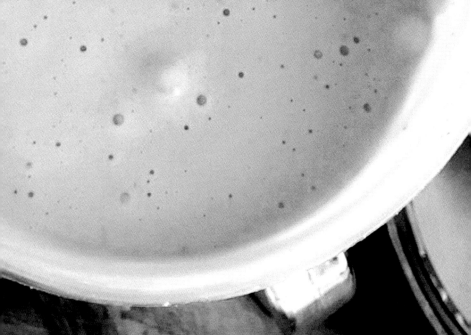

#smoothies

PEANUT-BERTA & JELLY

I would prefer to have pancakes with lots of butter and honey EVERY Saturday morning, but since that's not a realistic life goal, I defer to one of my favorite breakfast concoctions: The Peanut Butter & Jelly smoothie. It's simple and only requires 4 ingredients; you can alter the recipe slightly as you see fit. This recipe is EASY, quick and I usually ALWAYS have all the items on hand, frozen or fresh.

🛒 4 INGREDIENT **SHOPPING LIST**

1. 1 Banana (frozen)
2. 5 Strawberries (medium)
3. 1 Tbsp Natural Peanut Butter
4. 1/2 cup Water

optional
- Flax Meal - 1/2 Tbsp
- Ice cubes
- Protein Powder - 1/2 Tbsp

🍲 WHAT TO DO

Throw it all in the blender for about a minute or until smooth. I find the chillier the better – hence the frozen banana. This is great for breakfast, a snack or even post workout. Truly tastes amazing.

#PEANUTBERTAJELLY

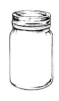

meal prep
5 MASON JARS (16 OUNCE) : REPEAT RECIPE X 5 : FREEZE UNTIL USE : DEFROST FOR 20 MINS : BLEND

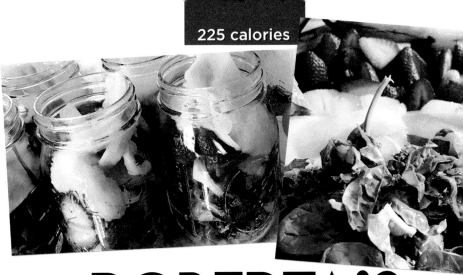

ROBERTA'S RAINBOW

I keep random but interesting colorful things in my refrigerator at all times. Super simple, healthy AND refreshing, smoothies like this have become my post workout staple. The sweetness of the mango offers a tangy kick.

4 INGREDIENT
🛒 SHOPPING LIST

1. 4 Strawberries
2. 1 half peeled Mango
3. Large handful of Kale
4. 1/2 cup Almond milk

🥣 WHAT TO DO

Blend with ice for about a minute or until smooth. Top with flax or chia seeds if you like. Gulp down, let me know you enjoyed it!

#ROBERTASRAINBOW

meal prep

5 MASON JARS (16 OUNCE) : REPEAT RECIPE X 5 :
FREEZE UNTIL USE : DEFROST FOR 20 MINS : BLEND

smoothies - SIMPLY TABBTASTIC

335 calories

BLU-BERTA
BANANA

No time? No problem! This smoothie is for the super time afflicted; grab a handful of everything! This smoothie is full of antioxidants, FIBER and protein.

5 INGREDIENT
🛒 SHOPPING LIST

1. 1 Banana (frozen)
2. 1 cup Blueberries
3. 1 Tbsp Peanut Butter
4. Large handful Spinach
5. 1/2 cup Almond Milk (Soy milk or Water)

🍵 WHAT TO DO

Throw it all in the blender for about a minute or until smooth and enjoy! I find the chillier the better – hence the frozen bananas. This is great for breakfast, a snack or even post workout.
Truly tastes amazing.

#BLUBERTABANANA

meal prep
5 MASON JARS (16 OUNCE) : REPEAT RECIPE X 5 : FREEZE UNTIL USE : DEFROST FOR 20 MINS : BLEND

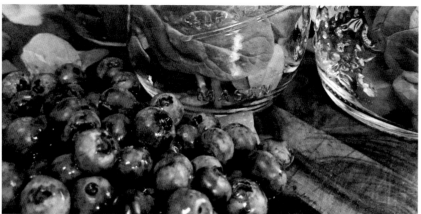

BERTA
BANANA-APPLE

Easy - because I usually have all these ingredients in the fridge or freezer. You can use kale or spinach, both taste slightly sweet and sour with the green apple. Pack the greens in - also creates a gorgeously green instagramable filterless color!

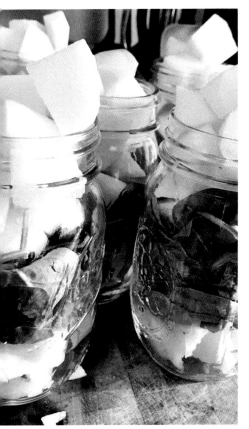

5 INGREDIENT
🛒 SHOPPING LIST

1. 5 or 6 Pineapple chuncks
2. Large handful Spinach/Kale
3. Medium cored green Apple
4. 1 Tbsp Natural Peanut Butter
5. Almond Milk - 1/4 cup

🍵 WHAT TO DO

Throw it all in the blender for about a minute or until smooth and enjoy!

Great for breakfast, a snack or even post workout.
Truly tastes amazing.

#BERTABANANAAPPLE

meal prep
5 MASON JARS (16 OUNCE) :
REPEAT RECIPE X 5 :
FREEZE UNTIL USE :
DEFROST FOR 20 MINS :
BLEND

smoothies - SIMPLY TABBTASTIC

300 calories

FALL BERRY BERTA

A smoothie without bananas! Though beloved, I don't always crave the overly sweet nature of them when they are ripe. The tartness of the cranberries paired with the light sweetness of the strawberries is a nice combination. Add a basil leaf and you get a bit of freshness.

5 INGREDIENT
🛒 SHOPPING LIST

1. 5 Strawberries
2. Handful of Cranberries
3. 1 cup of Spinach leaves
4. Handful of Raspberries
5. 1/4 cup of Almond Milk

🍵 WHAT TO DO

Throw it all in the blender for about a minute or until smooth and enjoy!

Great for breakfast, a snack or even post workout. Truly tastes amazing.

#FALLBERRYBERTA

meal prep
5 MASON JARS (16 OUNCE) : REPEAT RECIPE X 5 : FREEZE UNTIL USE : DEFROST FOR 20 MINS : BLEND

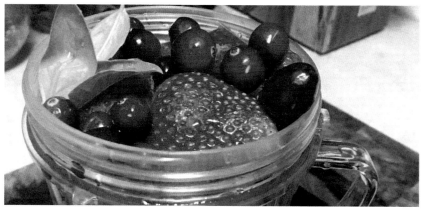

KIWI-KALE BERRY

Who knew Kale and Kiwi would blend so well together! Kiwi is another inexpensive but underutilized fruit, and like strawberries they are a little tangy and a little sweet. The Kale offers your daily greenery and the banana provides a dose of potassium.

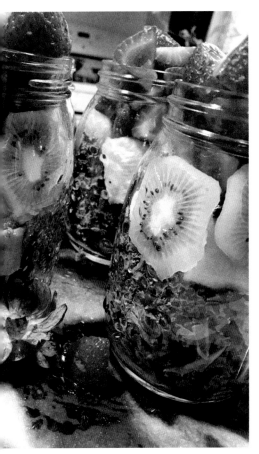

🛒 5 INGREDIENT SHOPPING LIST

1. Kale (2 large handfuls)
2. Half Banana
3. 4 Strawberries
4. 4 Kiwi slices
5. 1/2 cup water

🍮 WHAT TO DO

Throw it all in the blender for about a minute or until smooth. Great for breakfast, a snack or even post workout.

#KIWIKALEBERRY

meal prep

5 MASON JARS (16 OUNCE)
REPEAT RECIPE X 5 :
FREEZE UNTIL USE :
DEFROST FOR 20 MINS :
BLEND

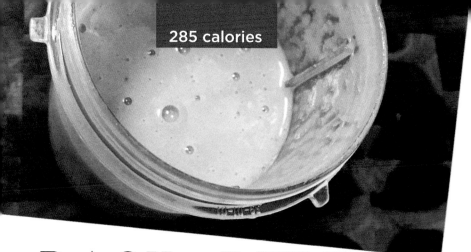

285 calories

BASIL-BERTA BANANA

*Another post gym smoothie – meal substitute idea.
This is a frequent favorite of mine. The texture of this smoothie
is silky velvet, the color VIBRANT and it smells heavenly. You
can also add half a green apple if you crave more sweetness.*

5 INGREDIENT
SHOPPING LIST

1. 1 Banana (ripe, frozen)
2. 1/2 Avocado
3. 2 handfuls Spinach
4. 4 Basil leaves
5. 1/2 cup Water

WHAT TO DO

Blend for a minute or until
silky smooth. Try adding ice
or 1 Tbsp of peanut butter!

#BASILBERTABANANA

meal prep

5 MASON JARS (16 OUNCE) : REPEAT RECIPE X 5 :
FREEZE UNTIL USE : DEFROST FOR 20 MINS : BLEND

smoothies - SIMPLY TABBTASTIC

BERTA'S BERRIES

Wonderful for midsummer when you can get 6 ounce packages of various berries as cheap as 2 for $5. It's simply berries and spinach, with added ginger for that extra kick. This smoothie is a little tart; if needed, you can mellow it with a teaspoon of natural peanut butter.

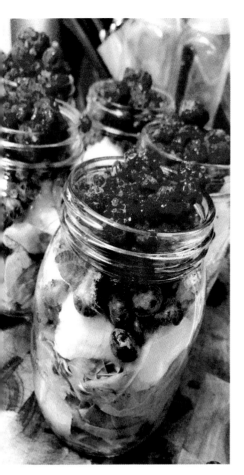

5 INGREDIENT
🛒 SHOPPING LIST

1. 10 Raspberries
2. 1/2 cup Blueberries
3. Large handful of Spinach
4. 1/4 inch Ginger
5. 1/2 cup water

🥤 WHAT TO DO

Blend for about a minute or until smooth. Try adding 1/2 Tbsp of peanut butter or flax seeds. ENJOY!

#BERTASBERRIES

meal prep
5 MASON JARS (16 OUNCE) :
REPEAT RECIPE X 5 :
FREEZE UNTIL USE :
DEFROST FOR 20 MINS :
BLEND

BEET ROOT BERTA

I dislike beets. I'm pretty confidant I went an entire decade without laying hands on one of these red roots. Beets taste earthy and are slightly sweet – I actually do enjoy the fresh aroma given once you cut them up. Try this receipe for a bit of beet, lots of flavor and a blast of fiber!

5 INGREDIENT
🛒 SHOPPING LIST

1. Half medium sized Beet
2. 1 small Green Apple cored
3. 1 ripe Banana
4. Large handful of Spinach
5. 1/2 cup of water

🍵 WHAT TO DO

Blend for about a minute or until smooth. Try adding with ice. ENJOY!

#BEETROOTBERTA

meal prep
5 MASON JARS (16 OUNCE) :
REPEAT RECIPE X 5 :
FREEZE UNTIL USE :
DEFROST FOR 20 MINS :
BLEND

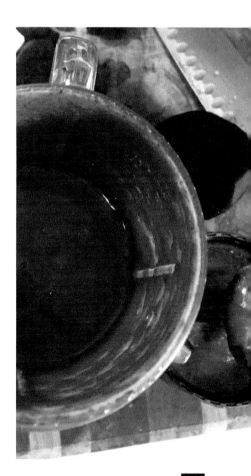

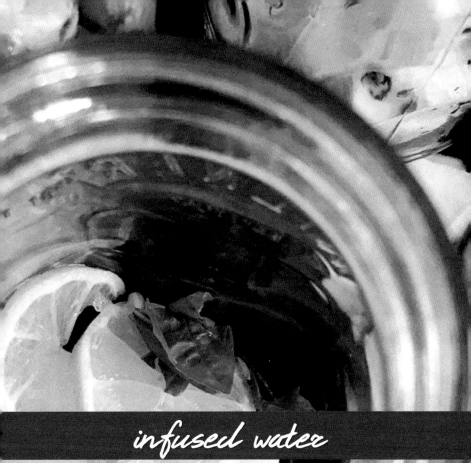

infused water

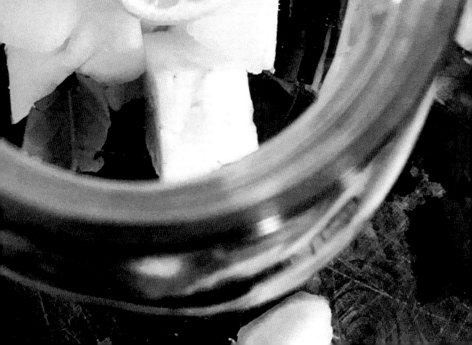

BASIL, LEMON, GINGER

INGREDIENTS
🛒 **SHOPPING LIST**

- **2 BASIL LEAVES**
- **2 LEMON SLICES**
- **1/2 INCH SHREDDED GINGER ROOT**
- **2 CUCUMBER SLICES**

🍵 **WHAT TO DO**

Place all ingredients in a 24 ounce mason jar.

MUDDLE FRUIT IN EACH JAR, juices should mix and fruits and vegetables should be slightly mashed. Herbs should be torn for best flavor and fragrant result.

Add ice. (optional)

Fill jars with filtered water.

Lid & refrigerate.

Enjoy up to 6 days.

meal prep
5 MASON JARS (24 OUNCE):
REPEAT RECIPE X 5 :
REFRIGERATE UP TO 6 DAYS

benefit Hydration | Refreshing | Detox |
Metabolism boost | Stress reliever

PINEAPPLE, BASIL, LEMON

INGREDIENTS
🛒 **SHOPPING LIST**

- **4 HALF INCH PINEAPPLE CHUNKS**
- **2 BASIL LEAVES**
- **2 LEMON SLICES**

🍵 WHAT TO DO

Place all ingredients in a 24 ounce mason jar.
For meal prep storage x5 recipe.

MUDDLE FRUIT IN EACH JAR, juices should mix and fruits and vegetables should be slightly mashed. Herbs should be torn for best flavor and fragrant result.

Add ice. (optional)

Fill jars with filtered water.

Lid & refrigerate.

Enjoy up to 6 days.

meal prep
**5 MASON JARS (24 OUNCE):
REPEAT RECIPE X 5 :
REFRIGERATE UP TO 6 DAYS**

benefit **Hydration & Detox**

infused water - SIMPLY TABBTASTIC

WATERMELON, LEMON, BASIL

INGREDIENTS

🛒 **SHOPPING LIST**

- **2 LARGE WATERMELON CHUNKS**
- **2 LEMON SLICES**
- **2 BASIL LEAVES**
- **1 JALAPENO SLICE**

🍵 **WHAT TO DO**

Place all ingredients in a 24 ounce mason jar.

MUDDLE FRUIT IN EACH JAR, juices should mix and fruits and vegetables should be slightly mashed. Herbs should be torn for best flavor and fragrant result.

Add ice. (optional)

Fill jars with filtered water.

Lid & refrigerate.

Enjoy up to 6 days.

meal prep
5 MASON JARS (24 OUNCE):
REPEAT RECIPE X 5 :
REFRIGERATE UP TO 6 DAYS

benefit Hydration | Refreshing | Stress relieving

LIME, STRAWBERRY, MINT

INGREDIENTS
🛒 SHOPPING LIST

- **2 LIME SLICES**
- **2 STRAWBERRIES**
- **1 SPRIG OF MINT**

🍶 WHAT TO DO

Place all ingredients in a 24 ounce mason jar.
For meal prep storage x5 recipe.

MUDDLE FRUIT IN EACH JAR, juices should mix and fruits and
vegetables should be slightly mashed. Herbs should be torn for
best flavor and fragrant result.

Add ice. (optional)

Fill jars with filtered water.

Lid & refrigerate.

Enjoy up to 6 days.

meal prep
5 MASON JARS (24 OUNCE):
REPEAT RECIPE X 5 :
REFRIGERATE UP TO 6 DAYS

benefit Hydration | Refreshing | Digestion | Reduces fatigue

LEMON, BASIL, GINGER, JALAPENO

INGREDIENTS
🛒 **SHOPPING LIST**

- 2 BASIL LEAVES
- 2 LEMON SLICES
- 1/2 INCH SHREDDED GINGER ROOT
- 2 CUCUMBER SLICES

🍵 WHAT TO DO

Place all ingredients in a 24 ounce mason jar.

MUDDLE FRUIT IN EACH JAR, juices should mix and fruits and vegetables should be slightly mashed. Herbs should be torn for best flavor and fragrant result.

Add ice. (optional)

Fill jars with filtered water.

Lid & refrigerate.

Enjoy up to 6 days.

meal prep
5 MASON JARS (24 OUNCE):
REPEAT RECIPE X 5 :
REFRIGERATE UP TO 6 DAYS

benefit Hydration & Detox

infused water - SIMPLY TABBTASTIC

18

BLACKBERRY, BASIL, LEMON

🛒 SHOPPING LIST

- 3 BLACKBERRIES
- 2 LARGE BASIL LEAVES
- 2 LEMON SLICES
- 2 CUCUMBER SLICES
- 1/2 INCH SHREDDED GINGER ROOT

🥤 WHAT TO DO

Place all ingredients in a 24 ounce mason jar.

MUDDLE FRUIT IN EACH JAR, juices should mix and fruits and vegetables should be slightly mashed. Herbs should be torn for best flavor and fragrant result.

Add ice. (optional)

Fill jars with filtered water.

Lid & refrigerate.

Enjoy up to 7 days.

meal prep
5 MASON JARS (24 OUNCE):
REPEAT RECIPE X 5 :
REFRIGERATE UP TO 6 DAYS

benefits Hydration | Refreshing | Detox | Stress reliever

used water - SIMPLY TABBTASTIC

ORANGE, BASIL, GINGER, JALAPENO

INGREDIENTS
🛒 **SHOPPING LIST**

- 1 ORANGE SLICE
- 2 BASIL LEAVES
- 1/2 INCH SHREDDED GINGER ROOT
- 1 JALAPENO SLICE

🍵 WHAT TO DO

Place all ingredients in a 24 ounce mason jar.

MUDDLE FRUIT IN EACH JAR, juices should mix and fruits and vegetables should be slightly mashed. Herbs should be torn for best flavor and fragrant result.

Add ice. (optional)

Fill jars with filtered water.

Lid & refrigerate.

Enjoy up to 7 days.

meal prep
5 MASON JARS (24 OUNCE):
REPEAT RECIPE X 5 :
REFRIGERATE UP TO 6 DAYS

benefit Hydration | Refreshing | Detox | Immunity boost

infused water - SIMPLY TABBTASTIC

CUCUMBER, STRAWBERRY, BASIL, GINGER

INGREDIENTS
🛒 **SHOPPING LIST**

- **2 CUCUMBER SLICES**
- **1 STRAWBERRY**
- **2 BASIL LEAVES**
- **1/2 INCH SHREDDED GINGER ROOT**

🍰 **WHAT TO DO**

Place all ingredients in a 24 ounce mason jar.

MUDDLE FRUIT IN EACH JAR, juices should mix and fruits and vegetables should be slightly mashed. Herbs should be torn for best flavor and fragrant result.

Add ice. (optional)

Fill jars with filtered water.

Lid & refrigerate.

Enjoy up to 7 days.

meal prep
5 MASON JARS (24 OUNCE):
REPEAT RECIPE X 5 :
REFRIGERATE UP TO 6 DAYS

benefit Hydration | Refreshing | Detox | Immunity boost

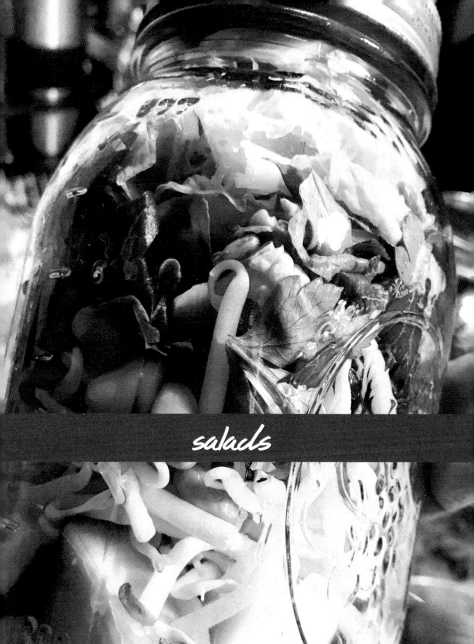

salads

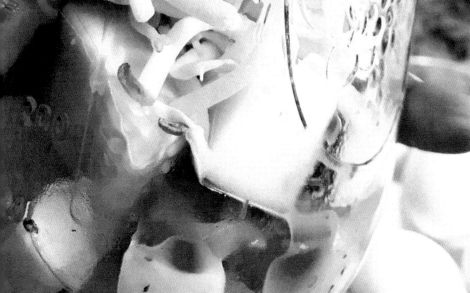

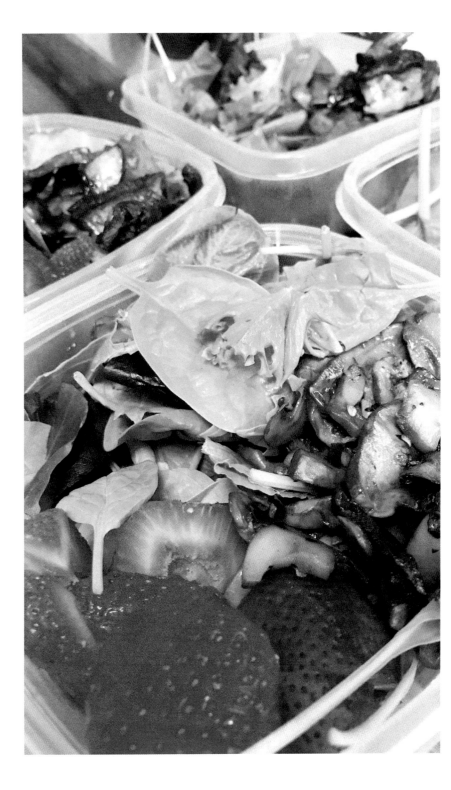

SPINACH STRAWBERRY MUSHROOM

🍲 WHAT TO DO

Spinach and strawberry, a longtime FAVORITE salad, but this time – in a jar! The advantage is that the jar makes a precisely portioned salad and the perfectly portioned dressing is already included. The ingredients are gorgeous. Remove and add as you see fit. Remember that the preservation is in the stacking; keep the wet with the wet and the dry with the dry or you'll end up with a soggy mess.

*be sure the dressing doesn't hit the sides of the jar, jars should be dry inside

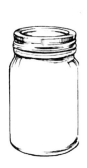

🛒 LAYERING LIST

1. Vinaigrette Salad Dressing (2 Tbsp per jar)
2. Mushrooms – 6 ounces (sliced)
3. 1 Cucumber (peeled & cubed)
4. 5 hardboiled Eggs – halved
5. Strawberries – 1 lbs. (sliced)
6. Spinach – 24 ounces
7. Gorgonzola – 3 Tbsp (crumbled)
8. Walnut pieces (handful)

meal prep

5 MASON JARS (24 OUNCE) : REPEAT RECIPE X 5
1. DIVIDE EACH INGREDIENT EVENLY 5 WAYS
2. LAYER THE INGREDIENTS IN ABOVE ORDER
3. REFRIGERATE (LOW SHELF OR IN CRISPER) FOR LUNCH OR DINNER

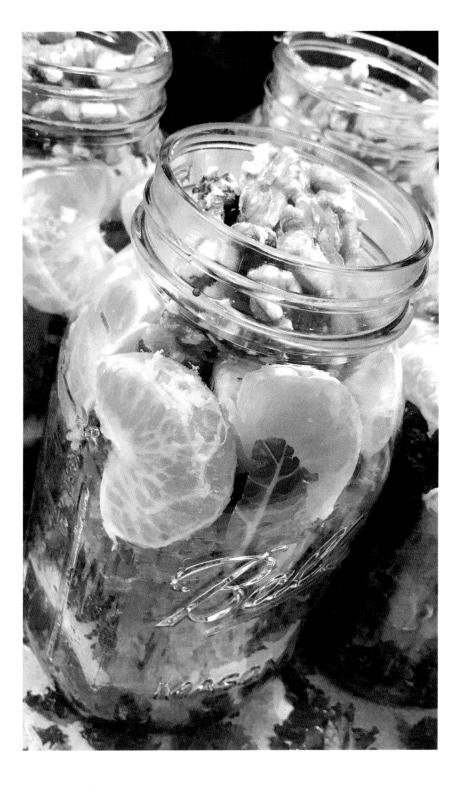

KALE & RED-QUINOA

Recently I discovered I LOVE red quinoa. I've used regular quinoa in the past but as a nutritional filler, not because I loved the taste. Red quinoa has a crunch to it, and has a nuttier taste than the regular. It also pairs perfectly with walnuts - they together elevate this salads flavor profile immensely.

*be sure the dressing doesn't hit the sides of the jar, jars should be dry inside

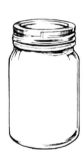

🛒 LAYERING LIST

1. Vinaigrette Salad Dressing (2 Tbsp per jar)
2. Red quinoa – 2 cups
3. Cucumber (sliced) - 1
4. Kale – 4 cups
5. Tangerine (peeled, pieces) – 4
6. Walnut pieces – 1 cup

meal prep

5 MASON JARS (24 OUNCE) : REPEAT RECIPE X 5

1. MASSAGE KALE WITH OLIVE OIL AND COARSE SALT
2. DIVIDE EACH INGREDIENT EVENLY 5 WAYS
3. LAYER THE INGREDIENTS IN ABOVE ORDER
4. REFRIGERATE (LOW SHELF OR IN CRISPER) FOR LUNCH OR DINNER

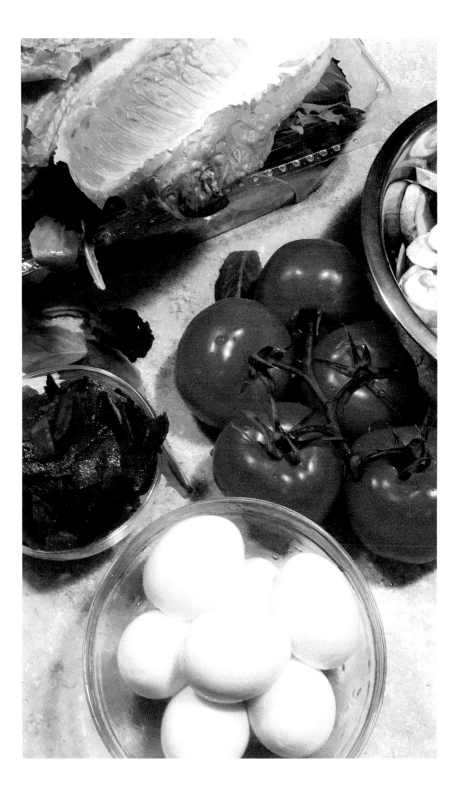

COBB JAR

I love great big messy cobb salads. More often than not, there are so many ingredients that the health factor is null and void. Cobb salad seems like a good idea, but really, it's just a tasty, filling farce; any healthy aspects of the salad are drenched in dressing and bacon! Here is my riff on a semi-healthy cobb salad. As filling as it is tasty for lunch, but probably at the bottom of the list of all my nutritionally inclined recipes. Layer as many veggies as you like as ordered below.

*be sure the dressing doesn't hit the sides of the jar,
jars should be dry inside

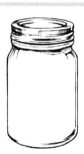

🛒 LAYERING LIST

1. Light Blue Cheese Vinaigrette Salad dressing
2. Mushrooms – 6 ounces (sliced)
3. Cherry Tomatoes – 6 ounces
4. 5 hardboiled Egg whites – halved
5. Turkey Bacon – 6 slices (chopped bite-sized)
6. Romaine Lettuce – 1.5 heads
7. Blue Cheese crumbles – 3 Tbsp

Avocado – 2.5 (optional)
don't jar / keep separate

meal prep

5 MASON JARS (24 OUNCE) : REPEAT RECIPE X 5
1. DIVIDE EACH INGREDIENT EVENLY 5 WAYS
2. LAYER THE INGREDIENTS IN ABOVE ORDER
3. REFRIGERATE (LOW SHELF OR IN CRISPER) FOR LUNCH OR DINNER

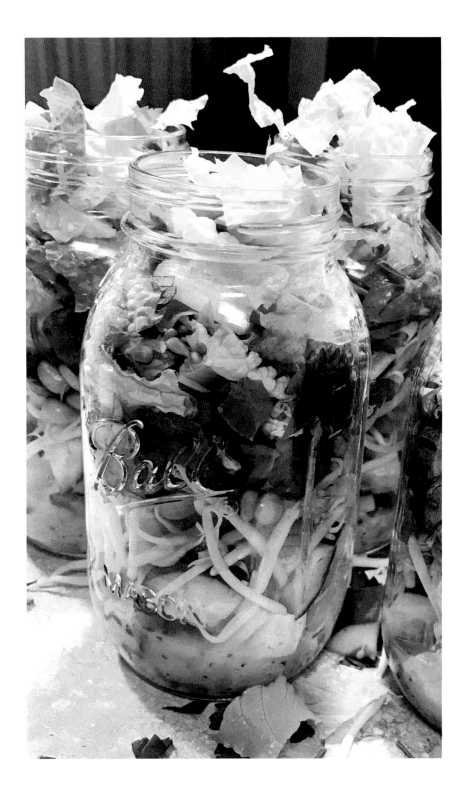

POWER HERB

I try to keep my recipes and meal prep very simple. The less ingredients the better, and I ALWAYS try to prepare meals from foods that can be found in your cabinet at any time. BUT, salads are often the exception. This Power Salad recipe is adapted from something I was recommended via Pinterest. I made some adjustments and Tabb'd it properly. Salads are the easiest preps I do – it only takes about 15 minutes from start to finish.

*be sure the dressing doesn't hit the sides of the jar, jars should be dry inside

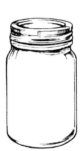

🛒 LAYERING LIST

1. **Vinaigrette Salad Dressing (2 Tbsp per jar)**
2. **Red Pepper flakes (to taste/optional)**
3. **Cubed extra firm Tofu – 12 ounces (optional)**
4. **1 Red Bell Pepper – sliced thin**
5. **1 Cucumber – chunked**
6. **Sprouts – 3 ounces**
7. **Shelled Edamame – 6 ounces**
8. **Sunflower Seeds – 2 Tbsp**
9. **Chopped Romaine lettuce – 1.5 heads**
10. **Chopped Parsley or Cilantro – 1 bunch**

meal prep

5 MASON JARS (24 OUNCE) : REPEAT RECIPE X 5

1. DIVIDE EACH INGREDIENT EVENLY 5 WAYS
2. LAYER THE INGREDIENTS IN ABOVE ORDER
3. REFRIGERATE (LOW SHELF OR IN CRISPER) FOR LUNCH OR DINNER

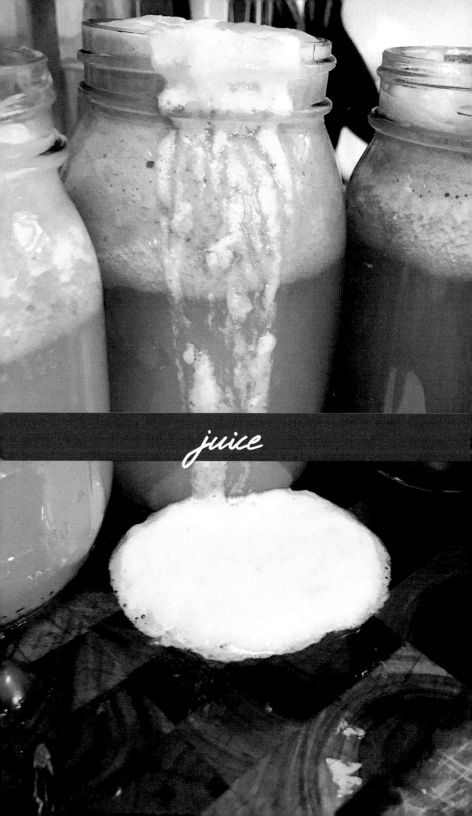

juice

THE **QUICK, DIRTY, WAKE UP**

A tangy, spicy alternative to regular green juice, this recipe is full of all sorts of good. If you need a WAKE UP or need an energy boost try the Quick & Dirty. The grapefruit and ginger play off each other while the apple mellows out the other flavors. This one will get you up and out!

🛒 SHOPPING LIST

- 2 Grapefruits
- 4 Celery stalks
- 4 Green Apples
- 4 Lemon
- 1 inch Ginger Root
- 3 Cucumbers

🍵 WHAT TO DO

Wash ingredients well. Juice entire fruit and vegetable – stems, skin & seeds.

OPTION 1:
as you juice each ingredient divide juice evenly into mason jars

OPTION 2:
juice everything all at once and dump into a large container, mix well then evenly distribute into mason jars

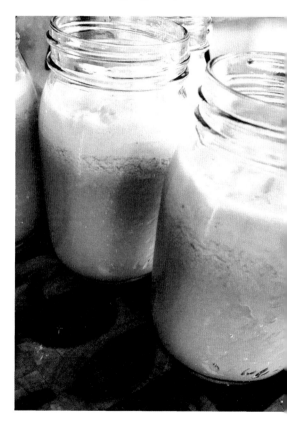

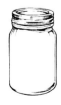

meal prep

5 MASON JARS (16 OUNCE) : DIVIDE EVENLY FILLING 1/2 INCH FROM TOP : FREEZE UNTIL USE : FOR LUNCH, REMOVE FROM FREEZER IN THE MORNING TO DEFROST : SHAKE WELL & DRINK

juice - SIMPLY TABBTASTIC

THE
RED WEDDING

The "Red Wedding" juice is named for the dominant BEETS! Despite all the fruits and veggies, the beet root overpowers all - and my kitchen... looks like a the Westrosi King of the North was murdered. Red wedding is slightly sweet and slightly spicy, but FULL of fiber and detox elements.

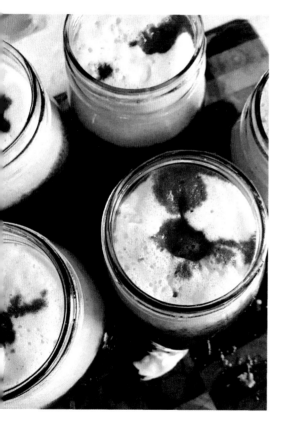

🛒 SHOPPING LIST

- **3 medium Beets**
- **5 Green Apples**
- **4 Lemons**
- **4 Cucumber**
- **1.5 inch Ginger Root**

🥣 WHAT TO DO

Wash ingredients well. Juice entire fruit and vegetable – stems, skin & seeds.

OPTION 1:
as you juice each ingredient divide juice evenly into mason jars

OPTION 2:
juice everything all at once and dump into a large container, mix well then evenly distribute into mason jars

meal prep
5 MASON JARS (16 OUNCE) : DIVIDE EVENLY FILLING 1/2 INCH FROM TOP : FREEZE UNTIL USE : FOR LUNCH, REMOVE FROM FREEZER IN THE MORNING TO DEFROST : SHAKE WELL & DRINK

juice - SIMPLY TABBTASTIC

THE **ANTI ORANGE**

Better tasting than boring orange juice and better for your immune system! I'm not the biggest fan of oranges, because I prefer sour over sweet, but orange and turmeric go great together. Turmeric is a little funky, but is loaded with antioxidants and anti-inflammatory properties. Basically, this juice is more magic in a jar.

🛒 SHOPPING LIST

- 4 Oranges
- 4 small Turmeric roots
- 4 Carrots
- 3 Apples
- 3 Cucumbers

🍲 WHAT TO DO

Wash ingredients well. Juice entire fruit and vegetable – stems, skin & seeds.

OPTION 1:
as you juice each ingredient divide juice evenly into mason jars

OPTION 2:
juice everything all at once and dump into a large container, mix well then evenly distribute into mason jars

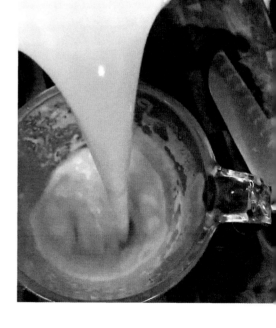

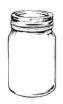

meal prep
5 MASON JARS (16 OUNCE) : DIVIDE EVENLY FILLING 1/2 INCH FROM TOP : FREEZE UNTIL USE : FOR LUNCH, REMOVE FROM FREEZER IN THE MORNING TO DEFROST : SHAKE WELL & DRINK

juice - SIMPLY TABBTASTIC

THE **SPICY GREEN LEMON**

A GREAT way to start a week of cleansing is with a delightfully spicy-sweet pick-me-up. The below is my green lemon recipe for cleansing and detoxing; virtually every ingredient has attributes that help detoxify and cleanse.

🛒 SHOPPING LIST

- 4 Celery stalks
- 4 Lemon
- 2 Jalapeño
- 5 cups of Kale
- 3 cups fresh Pineapple
- 4 Cucumbers

*Cayenne pepper to taste (I use 1/4 tsp per jar)

🍶 WHAT TO DO

Wash ingredients well. Juice entire fruit and vegetable – stems, skin & seeds.

OPTION 1:
as you juice each ingredient divide juice evenly into mason jars

OPTION 2:
juice everything all at once and pour into a large container, mix well then evenly distribute into mason jars

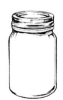

meal prep

5 MASON JARS (16 OUNCE) : DIVIDE EVENLY FILLING 1/2 INCH FROM TOP : FREEZE UNTIL USE : FOR LUNCH, REMOVE FROM FREEZER IN THE MORNING TO DEFROST : SHAKE WELL & DRINK

THE UNICORN: LIQUID MAGIC

True magic; each ingredient is GREAT for weight loss on its own, but combined, just imagine the possibilities! Weight loss, lowered cholesterol, improved digestion, great skin, nails & teeth also pain relief, reduced inflammation ... you MUST try this.

🛒 SHOPPING LIST

- 4 Green Apples
- 3 medium Beets
- 2 inch Ginger Root
- 3 Cucumber
- 3 Jalapenos
- 5 Celery stalks

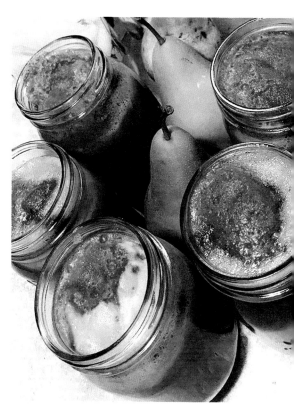

🫙 WHAT TO DO

Wash ingredients well. Juice entire fruit and vegetable – stems, skin & seeds.

OPTION 1:
as you juice each ingredient divide juice evenly into mason jars

OPTION 2:
juice everything all at once and dump into a large container, mix well then evenly distribute into mason jars

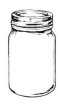

meal prep
5 MASON JARS (16 OUNCE) : DIVIDE EVENLY FILLING 1/2 INCH FROM TOP : FREEZE UNTIL USE : FOR LUNCH, REMOVE FROM FREEZER IN THE MORNING TO DEFROST : SHAKE WELL & DRINK

juice - SIMPLY TABBTASTIC

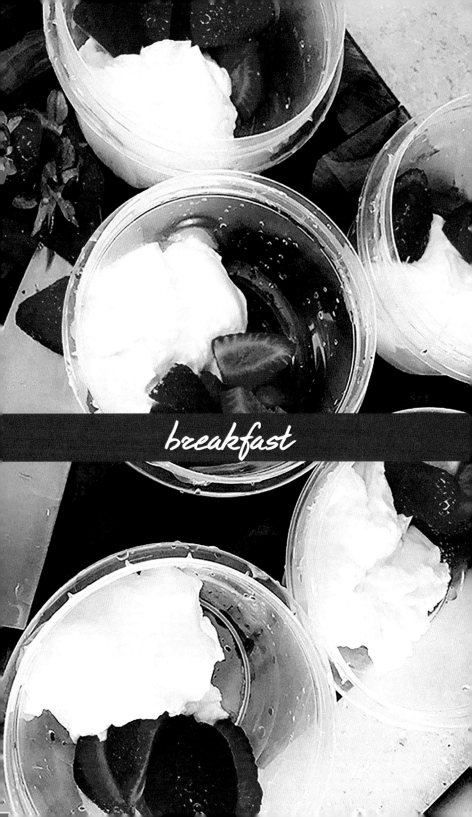

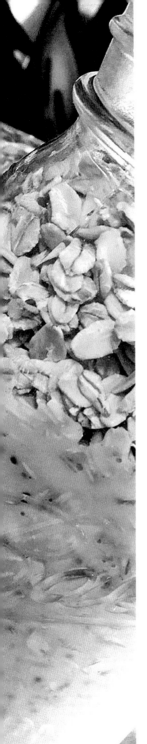

OVERNIGHT OATS

In the warmer months, overnight oats are a good example of a cool, fast and hearty breakfast. Oats have a filling effect and the berries offer a fresh aspect– these grab and go jars are just the right bit of both.

5 INGREDIENT
🛒 **SHOPPING LIST**

1. 1/2 cup Almond Milk
2. 1/2 cup Oatmeal
3. 1/2 cup Berries / Fruit
4. 1/2 Tbsp Vanilla
5. 1 Tbsp natural Honey

optional – chopped Nuts

🍲 WHAT TO DO

Add oats to mason jar. Add fruits, vanilla and honey, then pour in milk. Secure the lid and shake until mixed well. Refrigerate overnight. Top with nuts or a dollop of peanut butter.

meal prep
5 MASON JARS (16 OUNCE) :
REPEAT RECIPE X 5 :
REFRIGERATE UNTIL CONSUMED

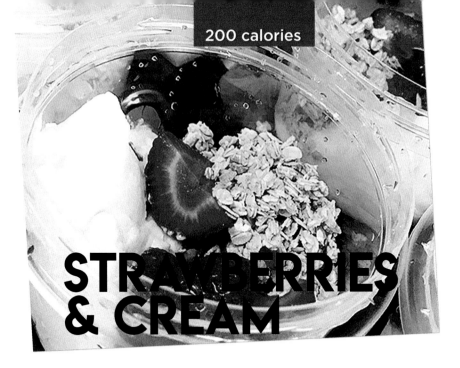

200 calories

STRAWBERRIES & CREAM

Super easy and only THREE ingredients. Plain Greek yogurt is a bit boring but full of protein – liven it up with a few fresh strawberries and some crunchy granola. My version of strawberries and cream stays fresh all week long, so it's wonderful for meal prep breakfast or a quick healthy snack.

4 INGREDIENT
🛒 SHOPPING LIST

1. 3 large sliced Strawberries
2. 1/2 cup plain fat free Greek Yogurt
3. 2 Tbsp all natural Granola
4. 1/2 Tbsp natural Honey

*optional 1 Tbsp Walnuts

🍱 WHAT TO DO

Easy; section each off the ingredients in air tight containers or mason jars.

meal prep
REPEAT X5 FOR BREAKFAST OR SNACK PREP :
REFRIGERATE UNTIL CONSUMED

breakfast - SIMPLY TABBTASTIC

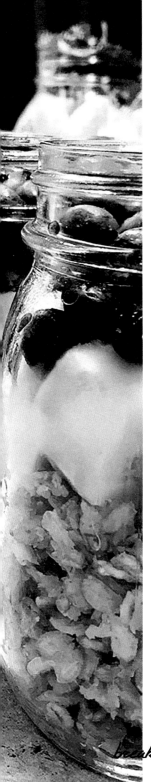

OATS & BERRIES

I grew up eating oatmeal. Usually Quaker "minute" oatmeal, filled with LOTS of sugar, butter and/or whole milk. Those days are long gone. My dad prepared the oatmeal soupy, I suppose to stretch breakfast on cold winter mornings. I hate soupy oatmeal, which is why I stopped eating it for half a decade or so. Fast forward to now, self--teaching as well as experimenting has brought me to a new appreciation for the health benefits of oats. Now try this!

3 INGREDIENT
🛒 SHOPPING LIST

1. 1/2 cup Rolled Oats/Oatmeal
2. 2 ounces fresh Fruit
3. 1/2 Banana

*optional 1 Tbsp Flax Meal

🍲 WHAT TO DO

Prepare the oatmeal as directed, let cool. Slice fresh fruit. Fill mason jars halfway full of oatmeal. Layer in the fruit. Sprinkle on a tablespoon of flax meal.

meal prep
5 MASON JARS (16 OUNCE) : REPEAT RECIPE X 5 : REFRIGERATE UNTIL USE : MICROWAVE JAR WITHOUT LID FOR 60 SECONDS

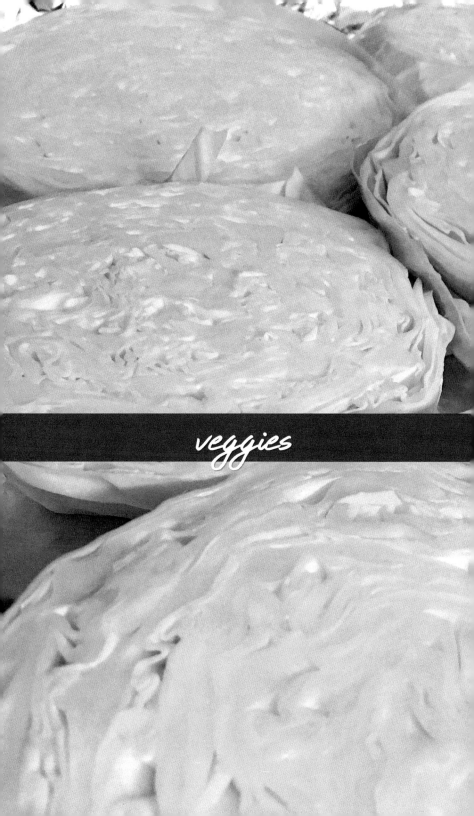

veggies

CABBAGE STEAKS

The first time I made these cabbage steaks I ate half of the cabbage head. Factor in that there are about 325 calories in a medium sized cabbage, that makes half a head a full meal in itself! You will save yourself many, many calories by prepping this flavor infused greenery for lunch instead of even a colorful salad.

5 INGREDIENT
🛒 SHOPPING LIST

1. 1 large head of Cabbage
2. 3 Tbsp Olive Oil
3. 6 Garlic cloves
4. Juice of 1 fresh Lemon
5. 1 tsp Salt

🍲 WHAT TO DO

I used a food processor to blend all ingredients – minus the cabbage BUT you can crush the garlic yourself and whip everything together with a fork.

The mix should be a little thick and perfect to spread, similar to butter.

Cut cabbage into 1 inch slices and lay flat onto lightly greased baking sheet.

Generously brush garlic mixture on top of each slice.
Bake at 375 for 35 – 45 minutes or until edges crisp.

benefit
VITAMINS K, C & B6, MANGANESE, FIBER & POTASSIUM

meal prep
**SEPARATE INTO 5 EQUAL PORTIONED CONTAINERS :
REFRIGERATE UNTIL USE : MICROWAVE FOR 60 SECONDS**

veggie · SIMPLY TABBTASTIC

AVOCADO SUNSHINE

Avocados contain GOOD fats and give plenty of energy to support a busy day. Furthermore, eggs are full of protein. With just 5 ingredients and 30 minutes of your time, you can accomplish a nutritious tasty meal. Just remember, everything in moderation!

5 INGREDIENT
🛒 SHOPPING LIST

1. 1 Avocado
2. 1 Egg
3. 1 Tbsp Freshly grated Cheese (I used asiago)
4. A dash of Salt
5. Red Pepper flakes to taste

🍲 WHAT TO DO

Preheat oven to 400 degrees.

Cut the avocado in half and remove the seed.

Scoop out a little extra avocado to make room for the entire egg (or just egg white).

Make sure the avocado is placed securely (slice off a piece of curved underside of the avocado if needed) on a baking sheet and add the egg into the scooped out indentation.

Sprinkle the grated cheese evenly then top with salt and pepper.

Bake for about 20 minutes or until the cheese is browned to your satisfaction.

benefit

VITAMINS C, E, K, OMEGA-3 FATTY ACIDS & NATURAL DETOXIFICATION

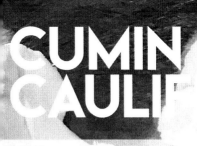

CUMIN CAULIFLOWER

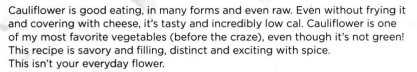

Cauliflower is good eating, in many forms and even raw. Even without frying it and covering with cheese, it's tasty and incredibly low cal. Cauliflower is one of my most favorite vegetables (before the craze), even though it's not green! This recipe is savory and filling, distinct and exciting with spice.
This isn't your everyday flower.

4 INGREDIENT
🛒 SHOPPING LIST

1. **2 whole medium Cauliflowers**
2. **2 tsp Cumin powder**
3. **2 Tbsp Olive Oil**
4. **Corse Sea Salt**

🍲 WHAT TO DO

Preheat oven to 400 degrees.

Cut the stem from the cauliflower and cut florets into 1 inch pieces and place in a bowl.

Mix cumin powder and olive oil well, toss the cauliflower in the mixture and fully coat.

Place cauliflower pieces flat on a foil lined tray or glass baking pan.

Lastly, sprinkle the coarse salt sparingly over the cauliflower.

Roast for 35-45 minutes turning once halfway through.

Bake longer for more tender result.

Cauliflower should be tender and browned at tips.

benefit
**VITAMINS C, K & B6 BOOSTS IMMUNITY
NATURAL DETOXIFICATION**

meal prep
**SEPARATE INTO 5 EQUAL PORTIONED CONTAINERS :
REFRIGERATE UNTIL USE : MICROWAVE FOR 60 SECONDS**

GREENS
KALE/SPINACH/COLLARDS

Super easy! A snack, a side or an entire meal – these greens WORK. Greens are truly a super food; highly nutritious, fat free and low calorie. Kale contains tons of vitamins A and K and is also one of the most nutrient dense foods on the planet. Spinach alike plays a part in reducing blood pressure and assists diabetes management.

4 INGREDIENT
🛒 SHOPPING LIST

1. **24 ounces - Kale, Spinach or Collard greens**
2. **1 Tbsp - Olive Oil**
3. **1 tsp - Sea Salt**
4. **Crushed Red Pepper flakes – to taste**
5.

🍲 WHAT TO DO

(Kale/Collards only) Wash fresh kale/collards in cold water. Massage with olive oil and sea salt, coating all of the leaves so that the color changes to a deeper green.

Place kale/collards/spinach in a deep skillet or wok lightly coated with olive oil and a tablespoon of water over medium heat. Sauté greens adding in a red pepper flakes to taste until slightly wilted (5-6 minutes).
Color will deepen but should still be vibrant.
Sprinkle a pinch of sea salt on top.

benefit
VITAMIN A & K, BLOOD PRESSURE REDUCTION & DIABETES MANAGEMENT

meal prep
SEPARATE INTO 5 EQUAL PORTIONED CONTAINERS : REFRIGERATE UNTIL USE : MICROWAVE FOR 60 SECONDS

veggie - SIMPLY TABBTASTIC

CANDY BEETS

Literally 3 ingredients. Used as a lunch dish or a side piece, these beets will have you beating with a new drum. Historically, I've never been a fan of beets, my father prepared them from a can, boiled and thickened with flour. Horrific. As an adult I thought they tasted like dirt, and while not entirely untrue, that earthy taste is one to be craved ever so often. I also love the beautifully colored juice beets produce and the magic that happens when you blend it with fresh ginger. The coconut oil really brings out the sweet earthy taste of the beets and the salt contrasts that perfectly.

3 INGREDIENT
🛒 SHOPPING LIST

1. **5 or 6 large Fresh Beets – spiraled OR chunked in half inch pieces**
2. **Sea Salt – 1/2 tsp**
3. **Coconut Oil – 2 Tbsp**

🍲 WHAT TO DO

Preheat oven to 400 degrees.

Put beets into a large bowl and drizzle on the coconut oil.

Toss the beets to make sure they are well covered then sprinkle on the salt, again tossing until evenly distributed.

Scatter beets evenly into a glass baking dish or foil lined cookie sheet.

Roast for 30-35 minutes, depending on preference you may want to bake a little longer for a crisper beet.

benefit
FIBER-RICH, ANTIOXIDANT, ANTI-INFLAMMATORY, AND DETOXIFICATION SUPPORT.

meal prep
SEPARATE INTO 5 EQUAL PORTIONED CONTAINERS : REFRIGERATE UNTIL USE : MICROWAVE FOR 60 SECONDS

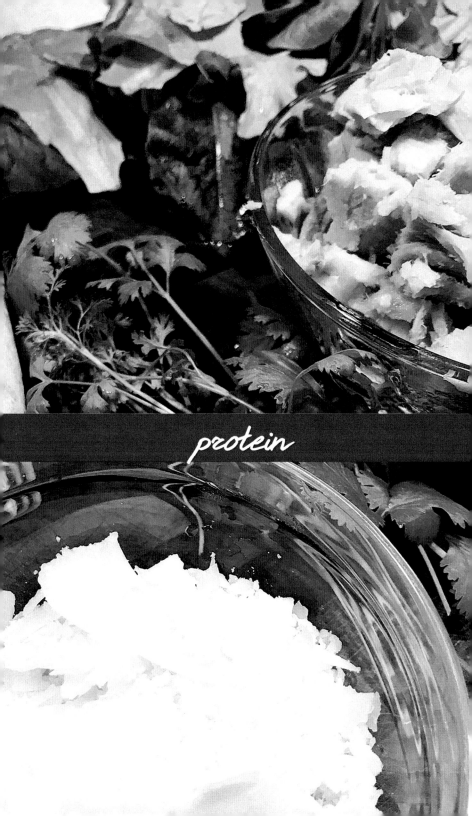

protein

TABB TUNA BURGERS

Tuna burgers are super easy, filling and great for a snack, lunch or dinner. Not to mention, tuna is full of protein, clean and low in calories – you can't go wrong. I enjoy these little burgers with avocado and cilantro.

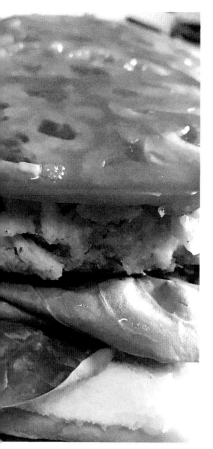

5 INGREDIENT
🛒 SHOPPING LIST

1. Solid White Albacore Tuna (in water) 4 cans
2. 3 Eggs
3. Bread Crumbs – 1/2 cup
4. 1/2 chopped Jalapeño
5. 1 tsp Salt

🍲 WHAT TO DO

Drain the tuna.

Mix all ingredients together well.

Form mixture into round patties, should fit the palm of your hand.

Heat pan or skillet to medium and coat with olive oil.

Once the pan is hot, drop the patties in cook until browned (about 4-5 minutes) on each side.

Yeilds 10 patties

meal prep
REHEAT : 45 SECONDS

SPICY-SWEET
SALMON
SKEWERS

Since I don't have a backyard or roof top to actually grill, I end up using my oven more than I should during the summer. In any case, I came up with a fun way to add protein and spice to my lunch or dinner with minimal work. Baked, spicy pineapple is always a WIN!

6 INGREDIENT
🛒 SHOPPING LIST

1. Salmon – 1 lb
2. 2 tsp Cayenne Pepper
3. Half Fresh Pineapple – cubed
4. 15 Cherry Tomatoes
5. 1 Tbsp Olive Oil
6. Corse Salt (to taste)
• 10 Wooden Skewer sticks

🍲 WHAT TO DO

Preheat oven at the broil setting.

Cut up the pineapple in square inch cubes, place in a bowl and toss with the cayenne evenly coating. Set aside.

Next cut the salmon into inch cubes and toss with olive oil.

Cut cherry tomatoes in half.

Create the skewers – you can use whatever combination you want; I was just careful to begin and end with the cherry tomato halves. Leave about an inch on each side of the skewers free.

Place skewers on a foil lined cookie sheet coated with oil (OR ON THE GRILL).

Broil for about 15 minutes or until tips start to brown/char.

meal prep

**LEAVE THEM ON THE SKEWERS
OR TAKE THEM OFF TO PACKAGE FOR LUNCH**

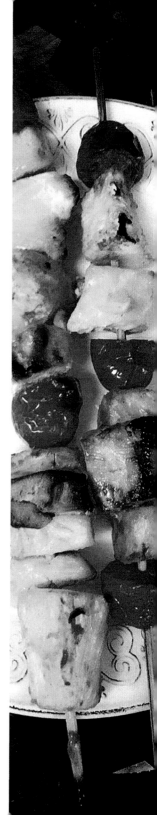

TUNA WRAPS

I grew up eating "tuna salad" on white bread with processed American cheese & Miracle Whip. The tuna was... regular tuna and in oil. Now that I know better, I do better. Here is my twist on a tuna salad sandwich, same concept but a healthier spin with big, bold flavors.

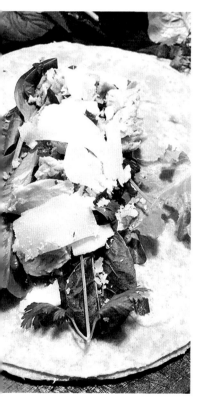

5 INGREDIENT
🛒 SHOPPING LIST

1. 1 Rye Wrap
2. **Spring Mix Lettuce**
3. **1/3 can White Albacore Tuna (drained)**
4. **Fresh Cilantro**
5. **1 Tbsp flaked Parmesan**

optional
- Lemon juice
- Red pepper flakes

🍲 WHAT TO DO

Stack all the ingredients in the wrap starting with the lettuce, and sprinkle on the lemon before you close it up (use a tooth pick to hold close if needed).

This is clean eating at its best and the epitome of filling, full of protein and oddly explosive flavors that pair amazingly well. Wonderful for lunch OR dinner.

meal prep
REPEAT STEPS X 5 :
STORE IN AIR TIGHT CONTAINERS UP TO 5 DAYS

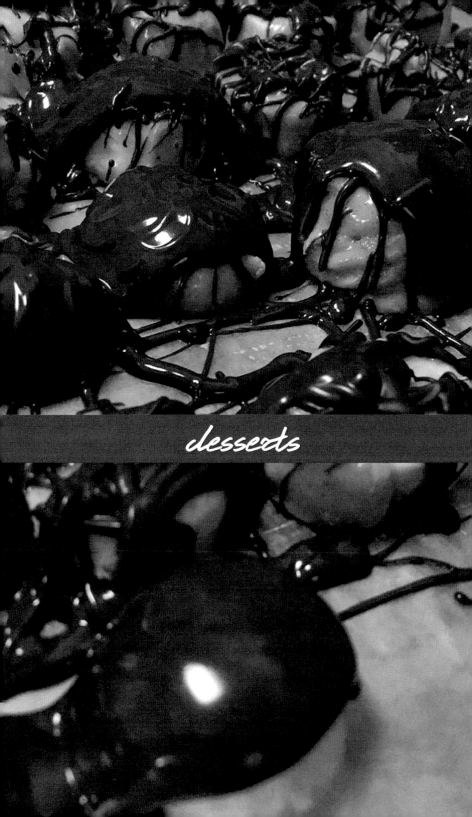

desserts

BERTA-BANANA NICE CREAM

So easy it's only 1 ingredient. All you need is frozen bananas and if you want to go crazy a few healthy toppers, like peanut butter, strawberries or nuts.

🛒 1 INGREDIENT SHOPPING LIST

1. **Banana - 1.5 (frozen)**

optional
- **Strawberries**
- **1/2 Tbsp natural PB**
- **1 Tbsp chopped Nuts**
- **1/2 Tbsp Cocoa Powder**

🍲 WHAT TO DO

Microwave frozen banana for 20 seconds. Or thaw for ten minutes on counter top.

Blend banana for about a minute and a half and enjoy! Nice cream is great for breakfast, a snack or even post workout. This potassium WIN, tastes suspiciously amazing.

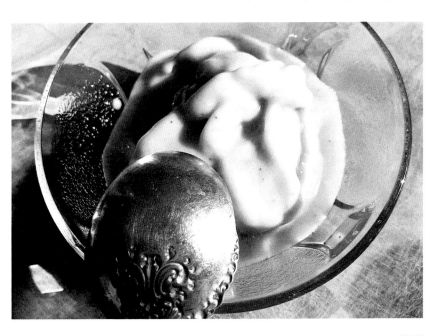

desserts - **SIMPLY TABBTASTIC**

FROZEN BERTA BITS

I came across a super easy dessert solution that also offers a bit of energy; thanks to the protein peanut butter. These bits are actually sinfully delicious ... but that's probably because I used too much chocolate. Don't make my mistake!

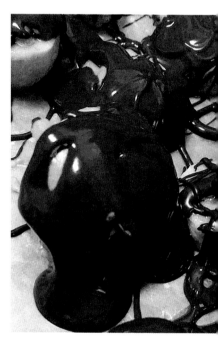

🛒 3 INGREDIENT SHOPPING LIST

1. **Bananas – 3**
2. **Dark Chocolate chips – 6 ounces**
3. **Protein or natural Peanut Butter (I used Nuts 'N More Toffee Crunch)**

optional - Sea Salt

🍫 WHAT TO DO

Cut bananas an inch thick. Lay them flat on a wax paper lined cookie sheet and drizzle on peanut butter (room temp, well mixed for best result). Put the peanut butter-banana mounds in the freezer for about an hour. While the bananas are setting, melt the chocolate using a metal mixing bowl over boiling water, mixing until smooth then set aside to cool. Once the chocolate has cooled to warm and the bananas are hard; drizzle (or dip) your desired amount of chocolate over the bananas and put them back in the freezer. Another hour should do well.

meal prep
SEPARATE 4 OR 5 SNACKS INTO PLASTIC BAGGIES, STORE IN THE FREEZER TO SNACK AT WILL.

BERRY BERTA BITES

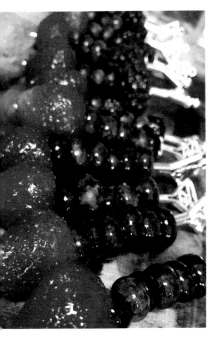

With as little as two ingredients and a little bit of patience, you can kill your sugar cravings. I like dessert, it's probably more accurate to say I LOVE desserts, and each night I think I deserve something sweet for just surviving the day. These yogurt bite thingies provide a deliciously light substitute, similar to a creamy popsicle. Prepare and keep a zip lock baggie full in your freezer for those extra intolerable days and live guilt free. Good for dessert or a snack.

2 INGREDIENT
🛒 SHOPPING LIST

1. Vanilla Greek yogurt
2. Berries
- Strawberries, Blueberries or Blackberries

*skewers or appetizer picks

🍲 WHAT TO DO

Use all the berries or just your favorites. Stack berries on skewers leaving about a 1/4 inch on both sides. Pour yogurt onto a plate evenly about half inch deep. Dip fruit skewers into the yogurt coating both sides (it will be messy). Place on drying rack or parchment paper. Freeze for at least an hour. Store in the freezer in air tight container or in zip lock baggies.

meal prep
SEPARATE 4 OR 5 SNACKS INTO PLASTIC BAGGIES, STORE IN THE FREEZER TO SNACK AT WILL.

step up your game

Your storage game! Not having the correct sized containers to grab and go, or mason jars to create all kinds of interestingly healthy recipes will devastate you. Growing up, no lid matched and aluminum foil was God. The solution is simple; hit up Amazon for very reasonably priced mason jars of any size and check out the dollar store (at the very cheapest) for at least two sizes of five set plastic containers. These are an investment of life.

get pinning

Join Pinterest and create a few boards of easy recipes to try. You can search healthy recipes for particular foods and develop ideas from other like-minded pinners. Pin ideas to these boards throughout the week to keep it interesting. Check out my Pinterest boards here: www.pinterest.com/therobertashow

budget

Hold yourself accountable. If you set a weekly food budget and you spend it entirely on meal prep ingredients, there is no room to spend buying lunch, breakfast or snacks during the work week. Also, you'll find that you'll save money, your ingredients for 5 days worth of food probably cost less than half than purchasing a healthy breakfast, snack and lunch for the week.

stay prepared

I always keep frozen fruit in the freezer. Whether it be ripened bananas, left over fruit from water infusing, or bags of frozen fruit I happen to see on sale. You can make a quick breakfast or lunch smoothie from these things if you can't get to the grocery store.

rule your SELF

In other words, be accountable. Don't waste the food you prepare and don't waste your money on extra food throughout the week.

be creative

Having a selection of foods and recipes that are interesting will keep you looking forward to each weeks meals. They probably all won't be perfect at first, but after a time you will recognize your favorites and build on rotating those.

life is preparation

Whether I'm planning my social calendar, workout days or meal prepping, faithfully I'm never at a loss for my time. Knowing that my time can't be given back, I try very hard to make each moment count.

One of my most favorite weekly rituals is Meal Prepping. Prepping offers me a sense of control and assurance that both my pockets and my mind appreciate. I sit aside at least 2 hours each week to prepare meals and snacks to last the week. I wouldn't call this an easy task, but consistently working this action into my weekly plan alleviates temptation and stress. In the end - there is no comparable feeling to having healthy foods at my finger tips whenever I need. **All I need to do is remember to grab something!**

set a time

Set a designated time during the week to prep. Persnally, I cook Sunday nights, but perhaps Saturday morning or Friday evenings work better with your schedule. I think it's important that you stick to the same time each week so you don't overbook yourself. (My meal prepping can be seen on my Snapchat or Instagram Story Sunday evenings @therobertashow)

check your calendar

Figure out what days you will need what meals for each week, you may need to exclude a meal or two for work lunches, social events and dates.

make a list

Go grocery shopping with healthy recipes in mind. Start with 2 veggies, 2 fruits, 1 protein and 1 carb. Depending on what you are prepping for the week, you may need to prepare multiple daily meals. Buy foods that stretch and that you can use in multiple recipes. Example: fresh fruits you can use in breakfast as well for snacks, fresh veggies you can snack on but also bake or sauté.

Also make a list of your FAVORITE healthy foods to combine with your grocery list (if you LOVE strawberries - get PLENTY of strawberries!)

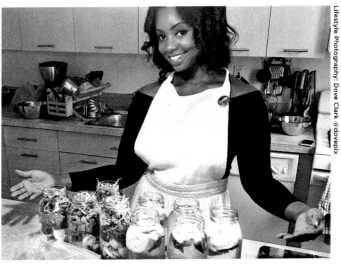

Lifestyle Photography: Dove Clark @dovepix

meal prep - SIMPLY TABBTASTIC

style your eating for YOU

75% of my weight struggle was overcome by healthier eating habits. Over a decade later, I still implement the dedication and discipline I used to lose half my size in weight. Lesson: The bases of eating healthy is to keep it simple. It's important to remember that foods that seem bad for you probably are. I put together foods that worked for me. Developing then KEEPING a consistent plan has helped me mentally and physically.

WATCH PORTION SIZES OR curate foods that are very low in calories & contain no fat, so that portion size doesn't matter (think FRESH & GREEN)

KEEP FRESH FRUITS AND VEGETABLES ON HAND - if it's always available, it will be easier to make the right decision when hungry (fresh produce for breakfast & snacking)

When shopping **don't give in to temptations**. MAKE A LIST – buy only the things included (also don't go to the store hungry)

Pick a time to stop eating in the evening - a few hours before you go to bed, 7 or 8 pm

DRINK LOTS OF WATER. Guzzling water is a great way to stay full, always keep a water bottle with you (get creative and try INFUSING!)

Don't drink sugars (these are empty calories) stick to black coffee & tea, fresh squeezed juices & smoothies only

No fast food AT ALL - remind yourself you no longer eat it

Don't eat to fill yourself up, eat to keep your energy up – eat to live, don't live to eat!

Don't deprive yourself, reward yourself on a good week with healthier dessert (see desserts section)

On holidays **DON'T take a second helping** OR leftovers

Try broiling, baking or grilling; you no longer fry anything

Buy lean meats – more expensive but it's worth it

Stay away from any foods in boxes (microwave dinners, rice & pasta sides)

Replace a meal with a smoothie

Keep a diet diary – daily record meals, snacks and times (the recorded process will either be inspiring or a lesson)

Download a free calorie tracking app to your phone – then USE the app

Weigh yourself no more than once a week – it's easy to start self-sabotaging and get discouraged, progress will not be instant
(pay attention to how you FEEL instead)

GIVE YOURSELF SIX WEEKS – be patient & STAY CONSISTANT.

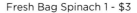
example weekly meal-prep shopping lists for one

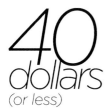

Fresh Bag Spinach 1 - $3
Blueberries/ Strawberries / Blackberries -$5
Quinoa (16 ounces) - $4
Lemons (4) - $2
5 Greek yogurt - $6
Peanuts / Nuts - $5
Fish or skinless Chicken Breast -$8
Eggs (dozen) - $3
Bananas (5) - $3
1 bunch Asparagus / 1lb Kale / 5 Sweet Potatoes - $4

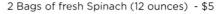

Oat meal (24 ounces) - $4
Carrot bunch - $3
Eggs (dozen) - $3
Bag of Kale (16 ounces) $3
1 jar Natural Peanut Butter $3
4 cans Albacore Tuna in water $6
Sugar Snap Peas / Edamame (6 ounces) $3
Lemons (4) $2
Large Cauliflower head $3
Almond Milk (1/2 gallon)$3
Bananas (5) - $2
Wheat Pita / Wheat wrap (6 count package) - $3
Chick Peas (1 can) - $2

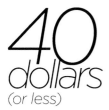

2 Bags of fresh Spinach (12 ounces) - $5
Cherry tomatoes (6 ounces) - $3
Eggs (dozen) - $3
Lemons (4) - $2
Apples (3 lbs) - $5
Mushrooms (6 ounces) - $3
Sunflower seeds - $3
Tofu (14 ounces) - $3
Bananas (5) - $2
Ginger - $2
dried Dates (6 ounces) - $4
Cucumbers (3) - $2
Greek Yogurt (16 ounces) - $3

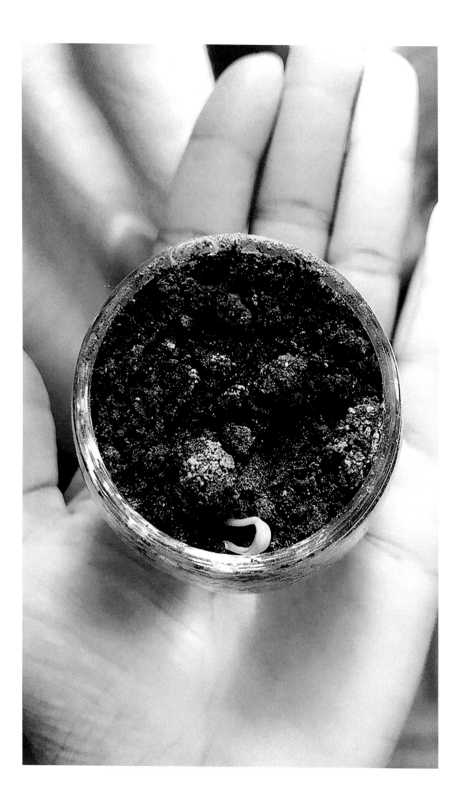

Made in the USA
San Bernardino, CA
01 January 2020

62538703R00038